Toenail Fungus Secret Weapons

Dan Kopen

www.NastyToenailFungus.com

The information included in this book is for educational purposes only. It is not intended nor implied to be a substitute for professional medical advice. The reader should consult his or her healthcare provider to determine the appropriateness of the information for their own conditions.

Contents

Introduction

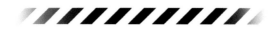

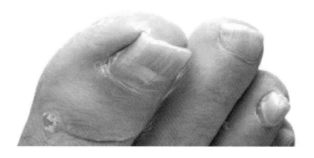

Toenail Fungus – I jokingly say it's just about the only thing that can survive an apocalyptic Armageddon. You probably know what I'm talking about. Sometimes it can feel like you'll need a NUCLEAR WARHEAD to finally get rid of your toenail fungus.

I know. I've been <u>exactly</u> where you are right now. And maybe I'm over exaggerating a tad bit with the whole nuclear bomb thing… I'm sure we both can agree that nail fungus is incredibly hard to kill, right?

Fortunately for you… You now have powerful *secret* weapons on your side… Which you can use to drop an ATOMIC BOMB on your nasty toenail fungus!

Hi, I'm Dan Kopen, a former victim of some really nasty nail fungus, and I'm about to show you exactly how you can ERADICATE your toenail fungus... By using a very unconventional approach that can yield some serious results.

Now before I even talk about all the different home treatments you can use... I want to make sure you understand exactly how nail fungus infections thrive and spread...

See most people falsely believe that you only have to directly attack the infected nail... using whatever nail fungus treatment they choose.

But the reality of the situation is... You not only need to apply treatment to your nails directly... But you also have to sterilize the environments you live in. Otherwise, you won't ever be able to fully exterminate your nail fungus problem.

So that means... Before you even begin using any of the treatments I'm going to suggest later on in this guide...

You need to first address the main problem...

The environment you live (or spend most of your time) in.

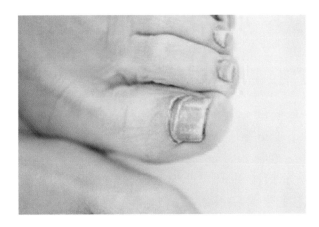

See in order for nail fungus to thrive, it needs the right conditions... And if areas in your house cater to those conditions, your entire living area can become a breeding ground for nail fungus.

In other words...Your infested living spaces can act as reinforcement "supply lines" for the fungus already on & under your toenails.

What that means is your nail fungus infection will not only get much worse over time... but it'll also get worse a lot faster!

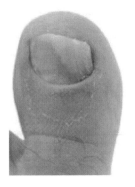
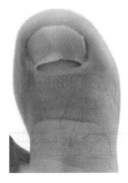
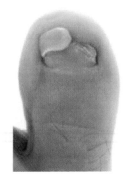

On top of that – you can also start infecting other people who walk anywhere in your fungus infested home. And because fungus can live for up to a month on its own in the right conditions...

Even if you do manage to completely kill your infection with a treatment... without addressing the route of the issue (your fungi infected living area)... You're guaranteed to get re-infected by many of the "rogue" fungus landmines scattered all around your house.

And here's where my "Toenail Fungus Secret Weapons" come into play.

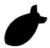

The secret weapons I'm about to teach you how to use can "NUKE" the environments that you spend most of your time in. And by doing this, you not only speed up the rate at which clear nail fungus under and around your nails, but also wipe out any remaining highly contagious spores that are clinging around in your house right now.

So with that said... Let's drop an atomic bomb on that toenail fungus of yours!

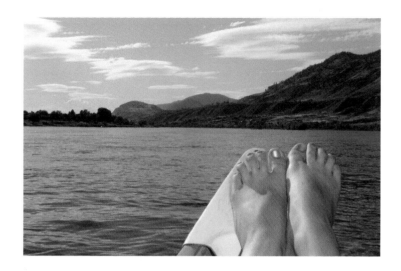

Now, since nail fungus thrives in warm, damp, and dark places... Let's start out by making your living area the exact opposite of that!

There are 3 areas of your house where nail fungus tends to congregate:

1. Your bedroom (You're more likely to be barefoot in your room)
2. Your bathroom (You're likely to be barefoot in the bathroom, and the shower provides moisture)
3. And your laundry room (socks & clothing that could contain nail fungus... + washing machine that can provide all the moisture fungi need)

First – Let's Take Care of the Moisture Problem – We Got to DRY Those Nasty Buggas Up!

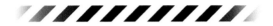

And if right now you're thinking that your house is perfectly dry… The fact that you have toenail fungus right now– and that it's spreading - is a good indicator that you could have a problem. So let's start by drying out the 3 key areas.

For this part, you'll need a dehumidifier (preferably 2). If you don't have a dehumidifier – I HIGHLY recommend you buy at least one ASAP.

The Eva-Dry EDV2200 is a good cheap dehumidifier that can cover a lot of surface area:

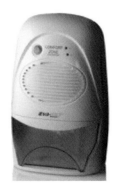

http://fungusbook.com/evadry

They are very quiet and if you can afford it, buy 2 of them. Look – nail fungus isn't a joke. If you truly want to get rid of it… and fast – you NEED a dehumidifier. Investing in one now is going to save you a lot of time and headache in the future. Since you spend roughly 8 hours each day in your bedroom, you'll want to put a dehumidifier in there.

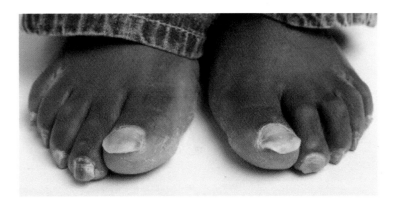

I know 1 dehumidifier doesn't seem like much – but this will make a HUGE difference with treating <u>any fungi in the area</u>, as well as help dry out your feet and nails to speed up the rate at which your nail infection is completely treated. If you can afford a second dehumidifier, place it in the bathroom you use most often.

After you take a shower, open the shower curtain an open the bathroom door. Then, activate the dehumidifier and keep it running all day.

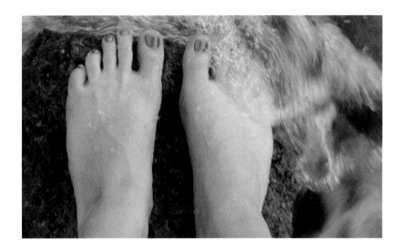

Now the last place you'll want to definitely dehumidify every few days is your laundry room. Think about this:

Your socks touch the toenail fungus all day long. You take off your socks and place them in your hamper. You take your clothes hamper and you dump the pile of clothes into the "needs washing pile."

The socks (covered with nail fungus) go into the washing machine. You start the washer, and wash your clothes. Now during this process of washing your clothes, not only have you contaminated all your clothes and the washing machine with nail fungus… But you've now served up a reliable source of moisture on a silver platter.

So you'll typically want to let your dehumidifier run for a couple of days at a time in there. You can alternate a dehumidifier between your bathroom and laundry room to save money.

And remember: dry air is your best friend.

Tip: if you can't afford a dehumidifier, at least open your windows and run some fans to help air your house out. It's nowhere near as effective as a dehumidifier, but it'll help.

Tip #2: You may also want to hit your living room and kitchen up every once in a while just to make sure nothing gets by!

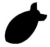

Next We're Going to FRY Us Some Nail Fungus!

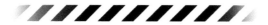

Nail fungus has the same weakness as vampires: LIGHT. Sunlight… and even light from a light bulb can work some serious magic on nail fungus.

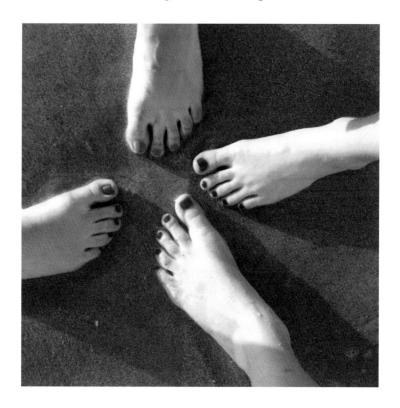

So I recommend when you leave for work each day… Leave the lights on in all the crucial areas of your house (or at the very least, your bathroom, bedroom, and laundry room). Keep your power bill in mind… And you don't really even need to go that crazy with it… Just leaving your lights an extra 12-16 hours per week can reap serious havoc on any nail fungus lingering around in your living areas!

Tip: Nail fungus is exceptionally vulnerable to UV light. Open your window curtains and let the sun shine down its powerful UV rays to fry nail fungus on contact!

Then We're Going to Freeze or BURN What's Left...

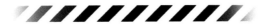

To continue bombarding your fungus infestation from multiple angles... It's good to change up the temperature of your attack!

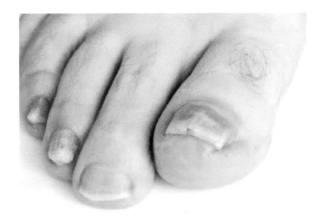

Since fungus THRIVES in warm environments, we can hinder it by either making your environment COLD or HOT. Depending on your geographic location, you may not be able to do this... If it's cold outside... turn off your house heater.... Or if it's hot outside... turn off your AC... Then open the windows of your house to absorb the outside temperature.

You're going to want to expose the nail fungus to either temperature extreme for a few hours at a time... a couple times a week if you can.

Not everyone can do this depending on the living situation, but this technique can help add a small boost to your treatment time. And just remember not to freeze anyone or anything to death!

Finish Off The Fungus By Spraying It With ACID

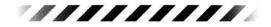

OK so you don't have to go to the acid extreme… But there are 2 common household items that can be turned into a spray that can melt away nail fungus on contact…

For bathroom tiling - use Bleach (be very careful with this around pets and children).

Get a spray bottle… Fill half with water/half with bleach.

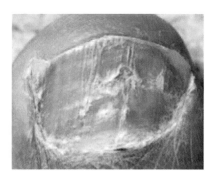

Once a week, you're going to want to spray your bathroom tub or shower with the water/bleach spray bottle mixture. Double spray any area in the shower that you stand in. You'll also want to spray the bathroom floor itself (tiles only – don't spray bleach on carpeting!)

After you spray, let it sit for half an hour, then wash away/mop up with water. <u>Be careful using bleach around pets and young children.</u> Whenever you bleach the bathroom, make sure you keep the door shut afterwards so no pets can wander in.

Important tip: DO NOT spray bleach on carpet or clothing. It will stain permanently!

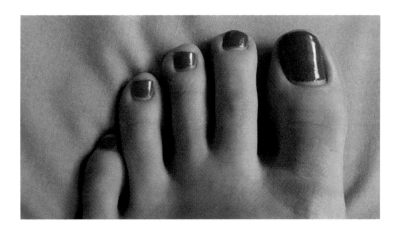

For carpeting – use tea tree oil!

Get a small bottle of tea tree oil from your local grocery store. Pour it into a spray bottle. Fill rest with water, and shake!

Tea tree oil is a powerful anti-fungal that can eat away at any remaining nail fungus landmines hidden within the fibers of your carpet.

Take the bottle and spray along common walkways and congregation areas (for example: in front of your living room couch). You'll also want to do this once per week during the course of your treatment.

Remember: DO NOT USE ANY BLEACH ON CARPETING!

The Ultimate Environment Nuking Tactic: Using Rapid Temperature Change On Key Clothing Items Infected With Nail Fungus

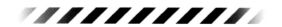

Fungus is particularly vulnerable to rapid temperature change: going from cold to hot… Or hot too cold within a short period of time…. Can decimate nail fungus on the spot.

Now unfortunately you can't really do this on a large scale… But you can use this tactic to nuke clothes items and bed sheets.

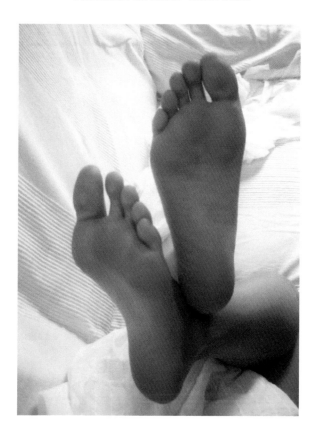

There are 3 things your toenail fungus comes in contact with every day:

1. Your bed sheets & comforter
2. Your socks
3. And your shoes

These key items can become so saturated with nail fungus… That it can be next to impossible to completely get rid of it. That's why it's important you address these items right when you start treatment.

So here's what you need to do:

Get 3 large zip lock bags and 1 black large kitchen-size trash bag (to fit your comforter in)... Take your socks and put them in 1 of the zip lock bags. Then take your shoes and place them in one of the other zip lock bags.

After that, take the bed sheets off your bed and shove them into the last remaining zip lock bag. Then, cram your comforter in the larger kitchen trash bag. Seal all the bags... Then cram them into your freezer for 8-12 hours straight.

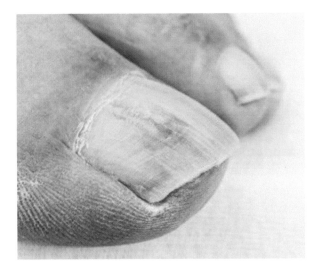

This freezing process REALLY damages the nail fungus (but usually not enough to completely kill every last bit of it). You may need to do this in multiple loads if you don't have enough room in your freezer.

Now immediately after you remove your clothing from the freezer…

You're Then Going To Rapidly Increase Temperature By Tossing Your Clothing Into Your Dryer

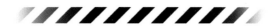

By taking your clothes out of the freezer… And then immediately run them through a dryer destroys nail fungus very thoroughly. Just make sure you don't accidently burn your clothing.

I suggest you check on the drying process every 5-7 minutes to make sure none of your clothes are dangerously hot.

Recommended Home Treatments To Directly Attack The Fungus Under Your Toenails...

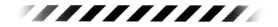

Here are treatments that you can apply from home that have worked for me:

The ZetaClear Toenail Fungus Treatment

I'm a HUGE fan of the ZetaClear for 2 reasons:

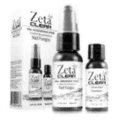

Overall Score:
★★★★★

"**Zeta Clear** worked remarkably fast considering the extent of toenail fungus..."

Buy ZetaClear Now

1. ZetaClear's dual acting formula attacks your nail fungus directly at the root underneath your nail, which can produce some serious results.

2. It's also EXTREMELY easy to apply. Most treatments require you to devote a good bit of time each to execute. With ZetaClear you can literally apply it in the morning within 30 seconds while you're putting your socks on.

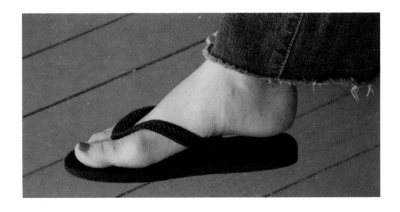

Combine ZetaClear with the other Toenail Fungus Secret Weapons you've already learned about… And you could possibly get your nails completely clear of nail fungus within 2 months. If you have a really bad infection spanning over multiple years, expect a 4 to 6 month treatment time. If you have multiple nails infected, you may want to consider picking up 6 bottles.

Go here for the ZetaClear website:

www.BuyZeta.com

If you get yours through the above link, you can **activate a super-fast shipping option** and possibly get your ZetaClear treatment kit in your hands within 24 hours.

Thermal Spa 49135 Professional U/V Gel Light Nail Dryer

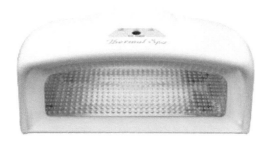

Use this UV nail light along with ZetaClear or any of the other treatments I recommend, and see your nail fungus melt away before your eyes.

Combining the UV light with ZetaClear can produce results equivalent to a professional laser nail fungus removal surgery... for 1/4 the price.

Get your UV light now – it's worth every penny:

http://fungusbook.com/thermalspa

Listerine Mouth Wash

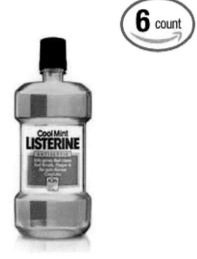

Listerine – known for its anti-fungal properties has been known to be a great home treatment for toenail fungus.

Simply get a Tupperware container large enough to fit your foot in, and fill it up with Listerine until your nails are entirely submerged under the liquid. Soak your nails for 30-45 minutes each day, and repeat for up to 2 weeks after your nail is entirely free of nail fungus. Replace liquid every 2-3 days.

Get a good deal for a Listerine 2 pack on Amazon here:

http://fungusbook.com/listerine

Vicks Vaporub

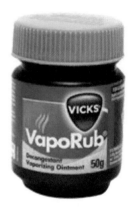

It sound strange – but Vicks Vaporub really does work as a nail fungus treatment.

Simply dab a good amount on a band aid, and place it over the infected area. Replace band aid and Vaporub, daily.

Get Vicks Vaporub shipped to your door from Amazon by using this link:

http://fungusbook.com/vaporub

A Cheap Alternative to a UV light – Small Magnifying Glass

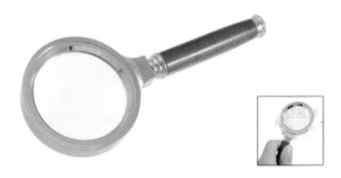

Focus light onto your nail fungus... And use the beam as a focused laser that will blast your nail fungus with concentrated UV rays.

Be careful with this – you're not trying to start a fire or melt your nail... you just want to do quick bursts of focused light.

If it feels hot, stop. Do this once a day to see some serious results.

This small magnifying glass will do the job:

http://fungusbook.com/magnify

Miconazole Nitrate 2 % Antifungal Cream

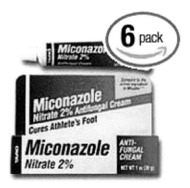

Anti-fungal creams are great to combine with treatments I've already talked about. You can even apply Anti-fungal cream after mid-day after your ZetaClear treatment.

Apply it using a Q-tip around the skin and infected regions of your nail.

Get powerful anti-fungal cream here from Amazon:

http://fungusbook.com/nitrate

Urine – Yes URINE!

Believe it or not your own urine is actually a natural nail fungus treatment. WWII soldiers would treat nail fungus they got in fox holes by urinating on their toes in the morning.

It's gross... but it can work. I don't think you need me to tell you how to do this!

Hydrogen Peroxide Footbaths:

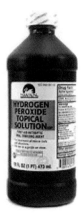

Simple household Hydrogen Peroxide has been known to work for nail fungus.

Simply fill a Tuba-wear container with enough hydrogen peroxide to cover your toenails. Soak for up to 30 minutes per day.

Get it cheap on Amazon here:

http://fungusbook.com/peroxide

Simple Household White Vinegar

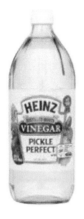

Common cooking vinegar is a proven treatment for toenail fungus. It does take a while for it to work if you use vinegar as your only treatment method… So I recommend you combine it with any of the other treatments I've recommended.

Simply fill up a container large enough to fit your foot with vinegar. Soak nails for 30 minutes daily.

Another way to apply this is by getting a cotton ball and soaking it with vinegar. Then using a band aid to secure it to your toenail. Put socks on over top, and go on with your day!

Get white vinegar cheap online through Amazon.com here:

http://fungusbook.com/vinegar

Barlean's Organic Oils Olive Leaf Complex, 16-Ounce Bottle

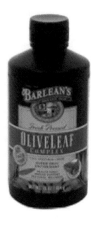

Olive Oil extract will help you keep your internal immune system strong... which can help get rid of nail fungus naturally. Some swear by this treatment.

Get Barlean's Olive Oil Extract Complex shipped fast from Amazon through this link:

http://fungusbook.com/organicoils

Types of Fungal Infections

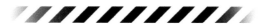

If you're interested in some more in-depth information on the causes and classifications of toenail fungus, this section will dispel some of the mystery behind this alien disease.

The technical name for toenail fungus infection is onychomycosis, and it's usually caused by skin fungi called dermatophytes. These dermatophytes actually hang around the surface of your skin quite often and they're usually kept in check by your body, but when the conditions are right (or more accurately, *wrong*) – meaning **moisture, darkness, and cramped or injured toes** – the dermatophytes can break through your body's natural defenses and colonize your toes like an alien invader! That's why it's so important to manage the conditions of your environment like I've talked about in this book before.

<u>There are four different major types of fungal nail infection:</u>

Distal subungual onychomycosis (DSO): This is the most common fungal nail infection and if you have toenail fungus, it's probably DSO. It invades the skin underneath the nail bed and this causes yellowing or whitening of the nail. Discoloration often starts at one or more parts of the nail and spreads from there.

Fragments of skin and nail build up between the nail and the nail bed and eventually the nail splits and cracks. The nail will also commonly thicken. It is a difficult condition to treat and, without intervention, can be lifelong.

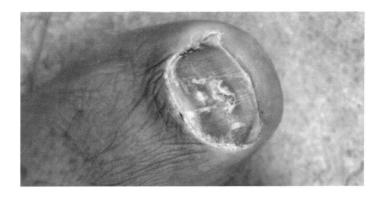

White superficial onychomycosis (WSO): This is the next most common fungal nail infection behind DSO. If it's not DSO, then it's probably WSO. It is caused by a fungal infection of the upper layers of the nail.

It causes a whitening of the top layer of the nail (white spots), and over time it will cover the whole nail. It is more easily treatable than DSO as it only affects the superficial layers of the nail as opposed to the deeper parts of the nail bed.

Proximal subungual onychomycosis (PSO): This is the least common fungal nail infection. It is quite rare and usually involves a compromised immune system. The fungal infection usually starts at the surface of the skin and burrows its way deep into the root of the nail. It can cause the nail plate to split from the nail bed.

Candidal onychomycosis: This is a related condition that essentially involves a yeast infection. It's more common on the fingertips, but can occur on the toes as well. It starts near the nail and attacks the skin nearby. Discoloration of the nail is common (brown, white, or green), and so are signs of infection like redness, swollenness, and tenderness of nearby skin. It can be quite painful, more so than the other types of fungal nail infection.

It's more common in people who immerse their hands or their feet in water more often than usual, or people who have experienced trauma or damage to their nails. A yeast infection in your toes or your fingertips might mean yeast infections elsewhere on your body, so if you suspect this is the case, a trip to the doctor might be in order.

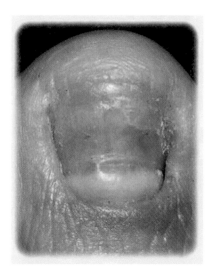

Age is a significant risk factor for toenail fungus. The older you are, the more likely you are to be susceptible to it. This is due to a large variety of health issues including weakened blood circulation and slower regeneration of nails. If you're younger, this doesn't mean you're out of the woods. It just means that *the older you are, the more you have to watch out.*

These types of fungal infections tend to affect more men than women. Family history can play a significant part in your risk level as well. If your family has a history of toenail fungus, then this should be a warning sign for you to take extra precautions and follow the instructions I've laid out in this book as carefully as possible.

Treatment for any forms of fungal infection can be a long and difficult process. New nail growth has to replace the old, infected parts of the nail, and this can take a long time. Having knowledge of the nature of your condition as well as some of the techniques laid out in this book for combating your infection will go a long way in helping you reach your goals.

Prevention

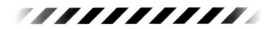

There are many steps you can take to help prevent fungal infections from spreading and coming back. Many of the home remedies I listed before in this book can work quite well, but for tougher, reoccurring infections, more serious secret weapons might be called for: <u>preventative techniques.</u>

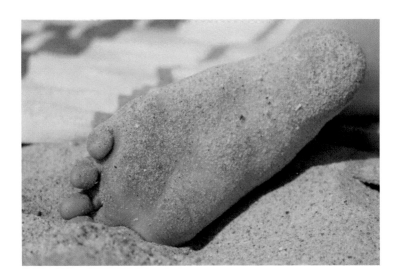

I talked about moisture before, but it bears repeating… One of the most important things you can do in combating fungal infection is being rigorous about **keeping your feet dry**. First of all, that means socks! Think about it… They soak up sweat and retain moisture almost like a towel wrapped around your feet. You need to change them often, especially if you sweat a lot or engage in frequent athletic activity.

There are different types of socks available to you. Clean cotton socks can work well. They're usually cheap and you can stock up on multiple pairs as you might need more than you're used to in order to get through the week. However, there are also synthetic socks, often available at athletic stores, that have moisture-wicking properties and they can be very effective as well.

If you work long hours, bring an extra pair to work if it's feasible – just be sure to properly contain your old socks (with a zip-lock bag) and wash your hands after handling them. If you're going out to the gym or the pool, always be sure to bring some spare socks!

Tip: Try out different types of socks to see what works best for your lifestyle in your efforts to keep your feet dry.

Your shoes can be a sponge for sweat and moisture as well, so it's important to keep them dry. For many athletic sneakers, you can toss them in the washer and let them sun dry to help keep them hygienic, though avoid using a dryer to dry your shoes as the heat can sometimes melt the rubber soles.

You can use vinegar on your shoes to kill fungus. You can get some vinegar here:

http://fungusbook.com/vinegar

Antifungal spray and powder can be effective as well. Use it on your feet as well as the insides of your shoes, but it's important to be consistent! The goal isn't to do it just once or whenever you feel like it. The goal is to build some of these preventative techniques into habits! And of course, as I mentioned earlier in the book, you can use antifungal cream as well, some of which you can find here:

http://fungusbook.com/nitrate

Continuing along the same thread, practicing good hygiene becomes very important when trying to prevent the spread and reoccurrence of fungal infections.

It might seem like a common routine, but cutting your nails while fighting or preventing fungal infections requires thought and care. You want to keep your nails short and trim to help prevent fungal growth, but you also need to be careful not to cut into the nail bed or cut into the surrounding skin either as this provides a pathway for further infection. These types of cuts provide a gateway for fungi and are completely counterproductive in our efforts to combat infection, so be extra careful when you clip!

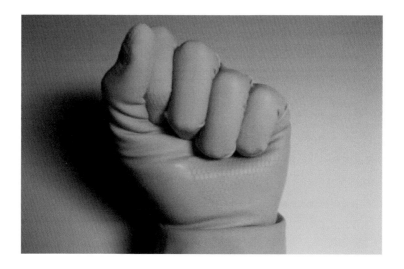

Your thoughts might be focused on your toes (understandably), but watch your hands! A prime way of spreading infection to and from your feet is through your hands. Rubber gloves can help protect you from the environment, so wear them if you need to do any cleaning, especially in areas with moisture. If your hands come into contact with an infected nail, wash them with soap!

Keeping your environment dry helps as well and using a dehumidifier like the one I mentioned before can make a real difference:

http://fungusbook.com/evadry

Also, it might seem like common sense, but **don't share anything that touches your feet with others.** That means socks, shoes, towels, floor mats, but even nail files and clippers! Unfortunately, when you're dealing with toenail fungus, you need to treat everything that comes into contact with your feet like a biohazard. Clean your nail clippers and anything else your feet come into contact with thoroughly between uses. It might get annoying, but this type of diligence is needed if you want to protect your environment and the people you live with from fungi.

And finally, if you're susceptible to fungal infection, consider laying off the nail polish. When you paint your nails, you can trap moisture between the polish and the nail plate, which is the opposite of what we've been trying to achieve this whole book. Avoid nail polish especially if you currently have a fungal infection as it will probably make things worse.

Remember, you're fighting a multi-front war. You want to use these secret weapons to directly attack the enemy like I've talked about so far, but also to shore up your defenses. These preventative techniques might seem tedious and inconvenient, but if you're serious about clearing your feet, protecting your living space and your loved ones, and keeping fungal infection from ever coming back, putting some of these preventative techniques into play will be necessary.

Athlete's Foot

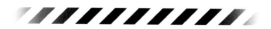

"Athlete's foot? I thought this was a book about toe nail fungus!" Yes, but did you know that athlete's foot is a fungal infection as well? That's right! Except instead of developing under your toenails, it usually develops in the areas between your toes. <u>The same fungus that causes athlete's foot is the source of some types of toenail fungi as well.</u> The two often go hand in hand as one source of fungal infection can cause further infection nearby.

If you notice any itchiness, burning, or stinging in between your toes, on the bottoms of your feet, or any cracking, peeling, or dryness of your skin around that area, athlete's foot might be a possibility, and it is often related to toenail fungus. Often both occur at the same time as the infection spreads so if you feel this is the case, it's important to take action!

The fungus that causes athlete's foot is often found in places like gyms, pool showers, gymnastics areas, and martial arts dojos, so if you frequent such places, be on the lookout. It is contagious and, like toenail fungus, can spread quite easily, especially in dark and damp environments.

There are a variety of over the counter and prescription treatments for athlete's foot, and a lot of the same tactics used to fight and prevent toenail fungus can be effective in combating athlete's foot as well.

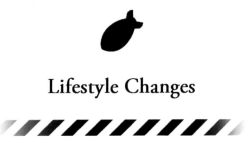

Lifestyle Changes

There are different lifestyle changes you can make to help you in your fight against toenail fungus. Sometimes home remedies aren't enough and you find yourself not making a dent in your current infection, or else you find yourself fighting reoccurring infections over and over again. This isn't the end! It just means you might need to be more aggressive with some of our secret weapons: specifically, <u>lifestyle changes.</u>

First of all, let's talk about footwear. Your shoes and your sandals are what separate your vulnerable feet from the moist, fungus ridden environment of the world all around, so in combating fungal infections, it's mandatory to take your footwear seriously.

Make it a habit of wearing footwear, not just in the usual circumstances. Wear something to protect your feet as much as possible, especially in public places like pools and locker rooms, breeding grounds for fungus. It can be tempting to go barefoot at times like the models on the magazines and the commercials on the beach, but take one look at the photos of fungal infections littered throughout this book and hopefully you'll realize <u>that it's more important to keep the big picture of your health in mind.</u>

There's a huge variety of footwear available to you, but you want to keep some general rules in mind. Your shoes should be roomy with space for your toes to breathe and wick moisture. Tight shoes damaging your toes can cause infections to spread or come back. A wide tip is crucial to preventing your toes from jamming together which can make the situation considerably worse.

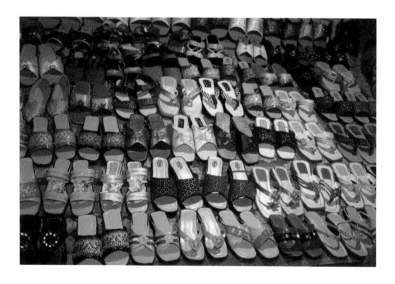

Open toed shoes and sandals are a great option to expose your toes to air and sunlight. Consider wearing shower sandals to help protect your feet from the dark and damp environment of your bathroom. If you do decide to use shower sandals, make sure to let them dry in between uses, otherwise they themselves can become a source of infection.

Tip: If you're a runner, increase your shoe size half a size to help reduce friction. Giving your toes room to breathe becomes doubly important during sweaty, athletic activity.

Improving your overall health in general can help you in your fight against toenail fungus. For one, stop smoking! It can affect your immune system and make the natural defenses of your body weaker, something you cannot afford when dealing with an enemy as stubborn and persistent as toenail fungus. If you've wanted to quit smoking but never gotten around to it, here's the perfect reason to give it a try!

A healthy diet might make a difference as well. Laying off the junk food and working on optimizing your nutrition will help with your overall body and you can use your toenail fungus as an opportunity to work on your whole-body health.

Another thing to consider, however, is that if you see any significant redness in your skin, it could be a yeast infection along with the fungus. Vinegar kills fungal infections and yeast infections as well. You can pick up some indispensable vinegar here:

http://fungusbook.com/vinegar

Adjusting your diet can definitely help with a yeast infection as well. If you think this is the case, avoid eating sugary foods as well as bread, cheese, and alcohol.

Of course, if you feel your situation is bad enough, you can consider seeing a doctor or a podiatrist. For especially stubborn cases, you may be given stronger prescription medications which can kill your fungal infection. For example, Lamisil is commonly prescribed to treat fungal infections. It's an oral pill and it can definitely do the job, but you can expect some possible side effects as well.

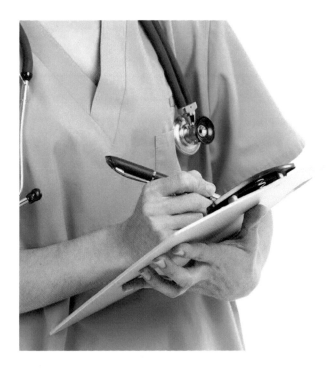

Your doctor might prescribe topical treatments like antifungal nail polish. You apply it to your infected nails every day, adding layer upon layer, and then at the end of the week, you wipe it all off and do it all over again. You continue this process for several months up to a year, and for some people it can make a difference.

And if all else fails, your doctor may suggest surgery, which can involve full removal of the infected toenail(s), thereby eliminating the infection completely. Of course, this is a drastic step and you should only consider it if none of the other treatments and techniques laid out in this book have worked, and only then on your doctor's or podiatrist's recommendation.

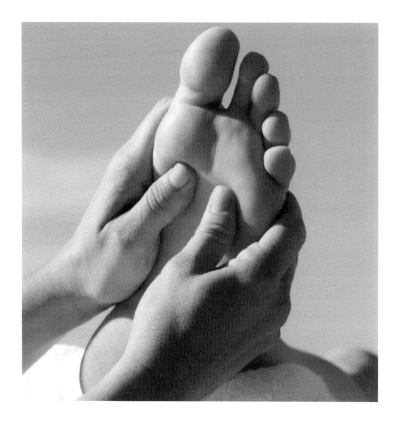

An important thing to keep in mind is that <u>toenails can take a long time to grow.</u> It could take several months or up to a year to clear up an infection using any of the methods described in this book. It's vitally important to be persistent with your new habits, because if you slack off halfway to your goal, you risk letting the fungus take control again and losing all your hard-earned progress.

In order to be truly successful in defeating toenail fungus and keeping it away for good, you'll probably have to make some lifestyle changes. That means not just quick-fix one and done treatments, but reorienting yourself and thinking more consciously about changes you can make in how you treat your feet and your environment on a daily basis as well as preventative measures you can take to fight and win some of the longer battles ahead.

Laser Surgery

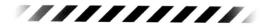

Like I talked about earlier in the book, toenail fungus is vulnerable to heat. Well, we can amp up the heat and throw it into overdrive with… lasers! That's right – we can use laser surgery to heat up your nail bed to temperatures hot enough to fry the fungus, but there are some drawbacks, so before you dive in, it's worth thinking it over.

The process involves first treating the infected toes with acid, and then treating them with a laser. However, it can be quite expensive – far more expensive than all the other options listed in this book. Your insurance may not cover it, so you might have to pay for the full treatment out of pocket.

Doctors who do laser surgery try to focus on the site of infection, but sometimes it can burn the nails and surrounding skin. It can be painful and that's something you need to be aware of going into the procedure. In addition, depending on the severity of the infection, follow-up treatments may be necessary which drives up the time and money required, as well as the pain you may have to endure.

However, for severe cases of infection where nothing you do is working, laser surgery is something of a "nuclear" option available to you if you can spare the expense, or if you just want to deal with the situation more quickly than some of the other lengthy treatments covered in this book.

<u>Before you plunk down the money for laser surgery, you should consider a technique I described earlier in the book</u> – namely, using a combination of ZetaClear and a UV nail light. You can potentially get laser surgery results at a fourth of the price with this combo "secret weapon" technique.

You can pick up some ZetaClear here:
www.BuyZeta.com

And you can pick up a UV nail light here:
http://fungusbook.com/thermalspa

The Key To Successful Toenail Fungus Treatment

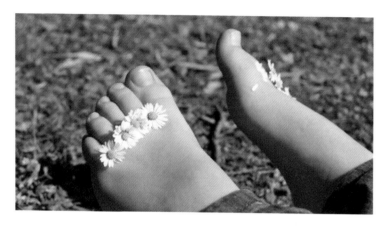

If you are truly serious about getting rid of your nail fungus, you must be consistent with applying treatment every single day. The moment you let up… it will start regenerating.

And remember: if you don't do something about your nail fungus now…

It's **<u>GUARANTEED</u>** to get worse.

And before long, you will start infecting other people who live in your house. If you think nail fungus is hard to get rid of now, just wait until everyone you live with gets it!

Good luck, and here's to you finally getting rid of your nail fungus for good!

-Dan Kopen

Video Reveals My Favorite Toenail Fungus Treatment Of All Time... And How You Can Use It... Along With Your Toenail Fungus Secret Weapons... To Clear Your Nails Within 6 Weeks...

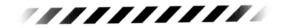

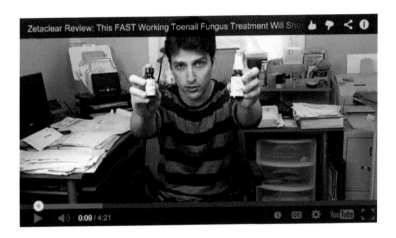

To watch this free video, go to:
www.NastyToenailFungus.com

Like My Book? Leave a Review On Amazon and Let Everyone Know About Your Opinion On Toenail Fungus Secret Weapons. Thank you! – Dan Kopen

Thank you for reading.

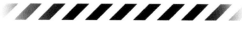

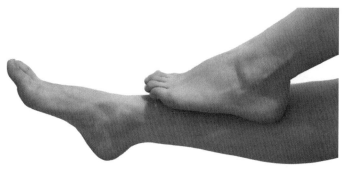

For more, you can visit
www.NastyToenailFungus.com

"Toenail Fungus Secret Weapons"
written by Dan Kopen @

www.NastyToenailFungus.com

CPSIA information can be obtained
at www.ICGtesting.com
Printed in the USA
LVIC04n1200280314
379359LV00007B/16

9 781494 427382